Mastering Prepping Equipment: A Guide for Outdoor Survival Enthusiasts

Table of Contents

Chapter 1: Understanding Prepping Equipment Essentials

Introduction

Embarking on an outdoor survival adventure requires careful planning, preparation, and the right equipment to ensure safety, comfort, and success. This eBook focuses on understanding prepping equipment essentials, enabling you to navigate the challenges and joys of wilderness living with confidence and ease.

The Comprehensive Guide to Outdoor Survival Living explores various prepping equipment categories, each packed with in-depth information, practical tips, and recommendations for high-quality, lightweight, and versatile gear tailored to your unique needs and preferences.

Navigation:

Learn how to choose and use the right equipment for effective navigation in various environments, ensuring you stay on track and reach your destination safely. Explore traditional methods like maps and compasses and modern technologies such as GPS devices and smartphone apps.

Fire and Heat Production:

Discover various fire and heat production methods and tools, including fire starters, matches, lighters, and alternative methods such as flint and steel sets or fire pistons. Fire and heat are crucial for outdoor survival, providing warmth, cooking capabilities, and a means of signalling for help.

Water and Hygiene:

Access to clean water and proper hygiene practices are essential for maintaining health and well-being during outdoor survival activities. Learn about portable water filters, gravity filters, life straws, water purification tablets, and essential hygiene items such as biodegradable soap, hand sanitizer, and toilet paper.

Food and Nutrition:

Find out about portable stoves, camping cookware, collapsible water containers, and food preservation methods such as dehydrated or freeze-dried food, mylar bags, and oxygen absorbers. Proper nutrition is vital for maintaining energy levels and overall health during outdoor survival activities.

Security and Protection:

Protect yourself from potential hazards and threats with personal protection devices, wildlife protection equipment, insect and pest protection, navigation and communication tools, first aid and medical supplies, and additional protective equipment.

By understanding prepping equipment essentials and gaining valuable insights into proper usage, maintenance, and storage for each piece of equipment, you'll enhance your knowledge and skills through first aid and survival training courses. The Comprehensive Guide to Outdoor Survival Living prepares you to tackle the challenges and joys of outdoor adventure with confidence. Embrace the journey, stay adaptable, and create unforgettable memories.

The Role of Prepping Equipment

Embarking on an outdoor survival adventure requires careful planning, preparation, and the right equipment to ensure safety, comfort, and success. This eBook focuses on understanding prepping equipment essentials, enabling you to navigate the challenges and joys of wilderness living with confidence and ease.

Prepping equipment plays a critical role in ensuring your well-being during outdoor survival activities, providing essential tools and gadgets to address various aspects of wilderness living. From navigation and fire-building to water and hygiene, food and nutrition, security and protection, first aid and medical supplies, power and lighting, and special considerations, prepping equipment enables you to overcome obstacles, maintain health, and enjoy your outdoor experience.

By investing in high-quality, lightweight, and versatile prepping equipment tailored to your specific needs and preferences, you can enhance your self-reliance, safety, and overall outdoor experience. Proper usage, maintenance, and storage of equipment contribute to your confidence and proficiency in various outdoor scenarios. Furthermore, enrolling in first aid and survival training courses can significantly improve your knowledge and skills, further preparing you for the challenges and joys of outdoor adventure.

Factors to Consider When Choosing Prepping Equipment

When selecting prepping equipment for your outdoor survival adventures, it's crucial to consider several factors to ensure you make informed decisions and invest in high-quality, lightweight, and versatile gear tailored to your unique needs and preferences.

Quality: High-quality equipment tends to be more durable, reliable, and effective, ensuring long-term performance and value. Prioritize reputable brands and well-constructed equipment that can withstand the rigors of wilderness living.

Weight and Portability: Outdoor survival activities often require long periods of travel and transport, making lightweight and portable equipment essential. opt for compact, lightweight, and collapsible gear, when possible, without compromising functionality or durability.

Versatility: Multi-purpose equipment that can serve various functions in different situations can be incredibly beneficial during outdoor activities. Prioritize items that offer versatility, enabling you to streamline your gear and maximize utility.

Ease of Use: Simple and intuitive equipment is often more accessible to learn, use, and maintain. opt for tools and gadgets with straightforward instructions and features that allow you to quickly become proficient and comfortable during your wilderness adventures.

Maintenance and Storage: Proper maintenance and storage of equipment directly affect its longevity and performance. Choose items that are easy to clean, maintain, and store, ensuring your gear remains in optimal condition for future use.

Cost: Balancing your budget with your equipment needs is crucial. While it's essential to invest in high-quality gear, it's also important to consider your financial constraints and prioritize items that offer the best value for their price.

Training and Skills: Before selecting equipment, consider enrolling in first aid and survival training courses to improve your knowledge and skills. Proper training will help you understand the functions and limitations of each piece of equipment, ensuring you make informed choices.

By considering these factors, you can choose prepping equipment that maximizes safety, comfort, and performance during your outdoor survival activities. Embrace the journey, stay adaptable, and create unforgettable memories with The Comprehensive Guide to Outdoor Survival Living.

Building a Comprehensive Prepping Equipment Kit

To build a comprehensive prepping equipment kit for your outdoor survival adventures, follow a systematic approach that considers essential items across various categories. Here's a suggested outline to help you create a well-rounded kit:

Navigation:

Topographic maps of the area

Compass

GPS device or smartphone app

Altimeter watch

Personal locator beacon or satellite messenger

Fire and Heat Production:

Fire starters (ferrocerium rods, magnesium blocks, etc.)

Matches or lighters

Flint and steel sets or fire pistons

Tinder (dryer lint, cotton balls soaked in petroleum jelly, etc.)

Water and Hygiene:

Portable water filter or gravity filter

Life straw or water purification tablets

Collapsible water containers

Biodegradable soap, hand sanitizer, and toilet paper

Food and Nutrition:

Portable stove and camping cookware

Collapsible water containers

Dehydrated or freeze-dried food

Mylar bags and oxygen absorbers

Spice kit and seasonings

Security and Protection:

Personal protection devices

Wildlife protection equipment (bear spray, electric fence, etc.)

Insect and pest protection (mosquito netting, bug repellent, etc.)

First aid and medical supplies

Additional protective equipment (helmets, harnesses, etc.)

Power and Lighting:

Portable power banks and solar chargers

Rechargeable batteries and battery chargers

Dynamo or crank-powered devices

Headlamps, flashlights, or lanterns

Special Considerations:

Specialized first aid kits or medical supplies (EpiPen, inhaler, etc.)

Satellite messenger or personal locator beacon

Portable water filter or purification system

When building your comprehensive prepping equipment kit, remember to consider the factors mentioned earlier, such as quality, weight and portability, versatility, ease of use, maintenance and storage, cost, and training and skills. This will ensure you make informed decisions and invest in high-quality, lightweight, and versatile gear tailored to your unique needs and preferences.

Embrace the journey, stay adaptable, and create unforgettable memories with The Comprehensive Guide to Outdoor Survival Living.

Chapter 2: Choosing the Right Shelter and Habitat Equipment

Introduction

Shelter and habitat equipment are critical components of your prepping equipment kit. They provide protection from the elements, a place to rest, and a base of operations for your outdoor survival activities. This chapter will explore various shelter and habitat options, emphasizing quality, durability, versatility, and ease of use.

Tents and Tarps

Tents and tarps are essential components of any outdoor survival kit, providing shelter, protection, and comfort during your wilderness adventures. Choosing the right tent or tarp requires careful consideration of various factors, including size, weight, materials, durability, and ease of use.

Tents:

Tents offer an enclosed shelter with walls, a floor, and a roof, providing a comfortable space for sleeping, storing gear, and escaping adverse weather conditions. Key factors to consider when selecting a tent include:

Size: Choose a tent that accommodates your needs while balancing weight and portability. Tent sizes are typically measured by the number of people they can accommodate. For example, a two-person tent is suitable for one or two people.

Weight: For backpacking or hiking trips, look for lightweight tents, as every ounce counts. Ultralight tents can weigh as little as 2 pounds, while lightweight options range from 3 to 5 pounds.

Materials: Choose tents made from durable, waterproof materials, such as ripstop nylon or polyester, with a waterproof coating (such as silicone or polyurethane) to protect against rain and condensation.

Seasons: Select a three-season tent for most outdoor survival activities, as they offer protection from rain, wind, and cold temperatures while remaining lightweight. For winter camping or extreme conditions, consider a four-season tent.

Design: Consider the tent's design, including the number of doors, vestibules, and interior pockets, to ensure a comfortable and organized living space.

Tarps:

Tarps provide a versatile and lightweight alternative to tents, offering protection from the elements and a flexible shelter solution. Key factors to consider when selecting a tarp include:

Size: Choose a tarp size based on your intended use. Common tarp sizes range from 5 x 7 feet to 12 x 16 feet, with larger tarps offering more coverage and versatility.

Material: Look for tarps made from durable, lightweight materials such as zillion (silicone-impregnated nylon), polyethylene, or ripstop polyester.

Shape: Tarps come in various shapes, including rectangular, hexagonal, and diamond-shaped, each offering different coverage and versatility.

Weight: Tarps are typically lightweight, with ultralight options weighing less than a pound and larger options weighing 2 to 4 pounds.

Accessories: Consider purchasing accessories such as trekking poles, tent stakes, or guy lines to enhance your tarp's functionality and versatility.

Ultimately, the choice between a tent and a tarp will depend on your personal preferences, the specific needs of your wilderness adventure, and your willingness to accept the trade-offs associated with each option.

By understanding the benefits and limitations of tents and tarps, you can make informed decisions and invest in the best shelter solution for your outdoor survival activities.

Hammocks and Bivvy Sacks

Hammocks and bivvy sacks offer alternative shelter options for outdoor survival activities, each with unique advantages and considerations. Understanding these options will help you make informed decisions and select the best shelter solution for your wilderness adventures.

Hammocks:

Hammocks are a comfortable and versatile shelter option, providing a cozy sleeping arrangement suspended off the ground. Key factors to consider when selecting a hammock include:

Size: Choose a hammock that accommodates your body size and weight, with options available for single or double occupancy.

Weight: opt for lightweight hammocks when backpacking or hiking, with ultralight options weighing as little as 1 pound and larger options weighing 2 to 4 pounds.

Materials: Choose a hammock made from durable, breathable, and quick-drying materials, such as ripstop nylon or polyester, with a strong suspension system (such as tree straps or ropes).

Design: Look for hammocks with built-in bug nets and weather protection (such as rainfly's) for added comfort and versatility.

Accessories: Consider purchasing accessories such as insulation pads, under quilts, or top quilts to enhance your hammock's warmth and comfort during colder conditions.

Bivvy Sacks:

Bivvy sacks, or bivouac sacks, are minimalist shelter options designed for ultralight backpacking and emergency situations. They offer a lightweight, waterproof, and breathable enclosure for sleeping bags, providing a compact and portable shelter solution. Key factors to consider when selecting a bivvy sack include:

Size: Choose a bivvy sack that accommodates your sleeping bag, with options available for mummy-style or rectangular bags.

Weight: opt for ultralight bivvy sacks, which can weigh as little as 8 ounces, or lightweight options weighing 1 to 2 pounds.

Materials: Look for bivvy sacks made from waterproof, breathable materials such as Gore-Tex, event, or Pretext Shield.

Design: Consider the bivvy sack's design, including the presence of a hood, zippers, and breathability vents, to ensure a comfortable and secure sleeping environment.

Accessories: Some bivvy sacks come with integrated bug nets or poles, providing additional protection and comfort.

When deciding between a hammock and a bivvy sack, consider the specific needs of your wilderness adventure, your personal preferences, and your willingness to accept the trade-offs associated with each option. By understanding the benefits and limitations of hammocks and bivvy sacks, you can make informed decisions and invest in the best shelter solution for your outdoor survival activities.

Sleeping Bags and Pads

Sleeping bags and pads are essential components of any outdoor survival kit, providing warmth, insulation, and comfort during your wilderness adventures. With various types, materials, and designs to consider, understanding these options will help you make informed decisions and select the best sleeping system for your needs.

Sleeping Bags:

Sleeping bags are portable sleeping systems designed to provide warmth and insulation in outdoor environments. Key factors to consider when selecting a sleeping bag include:

Temperature Rating: Choose a sleeping bag with a temperature rating suitable for your intended use, taking into account the lowest temperatures you might encounter.

Shape: Sleeping bags come in various shapes, including mummy, semi-rectangular, and rectangular. Mummy bags offer a snug, lightweight, and efficient heat-retaining design but may be less spacious than rectangular bags.

Insulation: Sleeping bags can use synthetic or down insulation. Down insulation is generally warmer, more compressible, and longer-lasting than synthetic insulation but is more expensive and loses its insulating properties when wet.

Materials: Look for sleeping bags made from durable, breathable, and quick-drying materials, such as ripstop nylon or polyester, to ensure the bag lasts and remains comfortable throughout your wilderness adventures.

Additional Features: Consider additional features such as draft collars, zipper draft tubes, and integrated hoods to enhance your sleeping bag's warmth and versatility.

Sleeping Pads:

Sleeping pads provide insulation and cushioning from the ground, enhancing your sleeping bag's performance and comfort. Key factors to consider when selecting a sleeping pad include:

Insulation: Sleeping pads can provide insulation through either air-insulated or reflective barriers. Air-insulated pads offer superior warmth and comfort, while reflective barrier pads are more lightweight and compact.

Thickness and Cushioning: Choose a sleeping pad with appropriate thickness and cushioning to provide adequate support and comfort.

Weight and Packed Size: opt for lightweight and compact sleeping pads when backpacking or hiking, with ultralight options weighing as little as 10 ounces and larger options weighing 1 to 2 pounds.

Materials: Look for sleeping pads made from durable, abrasion-resistant materials, such as ripstop nylon or polyester, to ensure the pad lasts and remains functional throughout your wilderness adventures.

Shape and Design: Consider the pad's shape and design, such as tapered or rectangular, to ensure it fits well within your tent or tarp setup.

When assembling your outdoor sleeping system, consider the specific needs of your wilderness adventure, your personal preferences, and your willingness to accept the trade-offs associated with each option. By understanding the benefits and limitations of sleeping bags and pads, you can make informed decisions and invest in the best sleeping system

Stoves and Cooking Equipment

Stoves and cooking equipment are essential components of any outdoor survival kit, allowing you to prepare hot meals, boil water, and cook over an open fire. With various types, materials, and designs to consider, understanding these options will help you make informed decisions and select the best cooking system for your needs.

Stoves:

Stoves are portable cooking appliances designed for outdoor use. Key factors to consider when selecting a stove include:

Fuel Source: Stoves can use various fuel sources, including canister gas, liquid fuel, alcohol, solid fuel, or wood. Consider the availability, cost, and weight of each fuel type when making your selection.

Output: Choose a stove with an appropriate output for your needs, measured in British Thermal Units (BTUs) or Watts. Higher outputs are ideal for boiling water quickly or cooking for larger groups.

Design: Consider the stove's design, including the number of burners, wind protection, and ignition systems, to ensure a functional and convenient cooking experience.

Weight and Packed Size: opt for lightweight and compact stoves when backpacking or hiking, with ultralight options weighing as little as 3 ounces and larger options weighing 1 to 2 pounds.

Simmer Control: Choose a stove with adjustable simmer control to regulate the heat output and avoid overcooking or burning food.

Fuel Efficiency: Look for stoves with good fuel efficiency, as this can reduce the overall weight and cost of your cooking system.

Stability and Durability: opt for stoves with stable and durable designs, as this can help prevent accidents and ensure the stove lasts through extended use.

Noise: Consider the noise level of the stove, as some stoves can be quite loud during operation, especially in a quiet wilderness environment.

Materials: Look for stoves made from durable, corrosion-resistant materials, such as stainless steel, titanium, or aluminium, to ensure the stove lasts and remains functional throughout your wilderness adventures.

Cooking Equipment:

Cooking equipment includes pots, pans, utensils, and other accessories needed for food preparation and consumption. Key factors to consider when selecting cooking equipment include:

Material: Choose cooking equipment made from durable, lightweight, and heat-resistant materials, such as stainless steel, titanium, or aluminium.

Design: Consider the equipment's design, such as nesting pots and pans or compact utensils, to optimize packed size and convenience.

Weight: Prioritize lightweight cooking equipment when backpacking or hiking, with ultralight options weighing as little as a few ounces and larger options weighing 1 to 3 pounds.

Accessories: Consider purchasing accessories such as pot grabbers, windscreens, or heat exchangers to enhance your cooking experience and maximize efficiency.

Cleaning: opt for cooking equipment that's easy to clean and maintain, with non-stick or anodized coatings to simplify the cleaning process.

Open Fire Cooking: Learn how to cook over an open fire using grates, grills, or skewers to prepare meals without the need for a stove.

Dutch Oven Cooking: Master the art of Dutch oven cooking, a versatile and efficient way of preparing meals using a heavy-duty, cast-iron pot over an open fire or stove

When assembling your outdoor cooking system, consider the specific needs of your wilderness adventure, your personal preferences, and your willingness to accept the trade-offs associated with each option. By understanding the benefits and limitations of stoves and cooking equipment, you can make informed decisions and invest in the best cooking system

Additional Considerations

When building your shelter and habitat equipment kit, consider additional components that can enhance your wilderness living experience, protect your gear, and improve the functionality of your shelter and habitat setup.

Groundsheets:

Groundsheets are protective coverings placed under your tent or tarp, providing a barrier between your shelter and the ground. Key factors to consider when selecting a groundsheet include:

Material: Choose groundsheets made from durable, waterproof, and lightweight materials, such as ripstop nylon or polyester, with a waterproof coating (such as silicone or polyurethane).

Size: Select a groundsheet that is slightly larger than your tent or tarp footprint, ensuring adequate coverage and protection.

Weight: opt for lightweight groundsheets when backpacking or hiking, with ultralight options weighing as little as 5 ounces and larger options weighing 1 to 2 pounds.

Repair Kits:

Repair kits are essential for addressing any tears or damage to your shelter and habitat equipment during your wilderness adventures. Key components to include in your repair kit are:

Tent and Tarp Patches: Pre-cut adhesive patches or repair tape designed for repairing holes or tears in tents and tarps.

Seam Sealant: Tube-based sealant for repairing and reinforcing seams on tents, tarps, or rainwear.

Zipper Repair Tools: Small pliers or other tools for repairing broken zippers on tents, jackets, or sleeping bags.

Duct Tape: Versatile, strong adhesive tape for securing and reinforcing repairs.

Sewing Needles and Thread: Hand-sewing supplies for more permanent repairs.

Stakes and Guy Lines:

Stakes and guy lines are essential for securing your shelter and habitat equipment in windy conditions, ensuring stability and safety. Key factors to consider when selecting stakes and guy lines include:

Material: Choose stakes and guy lines made from durable, lightweight materials, such as aluminium or titanium, to minimize weight and maximize lifespan.

Design: opt for stakes with a stable and secure design, such as a Y-beam or shepherd's hook, and guy lines with reflective features for easy visibility in low-light conditions.

Weight: Consider the weight of stakes and guy lines, with ultralight options weighing as little as 0.1 ounces per stake and lightweight guy lines weighing 1 to 2 ounces per 50 feet.

Storage: Look for stakes and guy lines that are compact and easy to store, with carrying cases or stuff sacks included.

Chapter 3: Navigation and Communication Tools for Preppers

Introduction

Effective navigation and communication are essential for outdoor survival and safety. This chapter will explore various navigation and communication tools to help you stay informed, connected, and on track during your wilderness adventures.

Maps and Compasses

Maps and compasses are fundamental navigation tools for any outdoor enthusiast. Familiarizing yourself with these essential navigation aids and understanding how to use them effectively will significantly enhance your ability to explore and navigate the wilderness with confidence.

Maps:

Topographic maps are detailed, graphical representations of the Earth's surface, providing valuable information about terrain features, elevation, and landmarks. Key aspects to consider when using topographic maps include:

Contour Lines: Contour lines represent lines of equal elevation, with the space between lines indicating the steepness of the terrain. Familiarize yourself with the contour interval (the vertical distance between contour lines) to understand the terrain's relative steepness or flatness.

Terrain Features: Identify and understand the various terrain features represented on the map, such as valleys, ridges, hills, and saddles.

Scale: Understand the map's scale, which indicates the relationship between distances on the map and their real-world counterparts. Choose maps with an appropriate scale for your wilderness adventure, balancing the level of detail with the overall map size and weight.

Landmarks: Locate and utilize landmarks, such as natural features (e.g., mountains, rivers, and forests) or man-made structures (e.g., buildings, roads, and trails), to assist with navigation and orientation.

Compasses:

A compass is a magnetic device that indicates direction relative to the Earth's magnetic field. Key components and aspects to consider when using a compass include:

Direction of Travel Arrow: The direction of travel arrow is a fixed, arrow-shaped indicator on the compass baseplate, pointing in the direction you want to travel.

Degree Dial or Azimuth Ring: The degree dial or azimuth ring is a rotating bezel surrounding the compass housing, displaying the 360-degree range of magnetic directions.

Magnetic Needle: The magnetic needle, typically red, points to the Earth's magnetic north pole. Align the magnetic needle with the compass's orienting arrow or lines to ensure accurate navigation.

Declination Adjustment: Declination is the difference between magnetic north and true north. Adjust your compass for declination by either adding or subtracting the declination value (depending on the direction of the offset) to the magnetic bearing to obtain the true bearing.

Clinometer: A clinometer is a feature found on some compasses, used to measure the angle of a slope or the height of an object.

Practice using a compass to navigate by aligning it with your map, taking bearings, and following the desired bearings to reach your destination. Familiarize yourself with magnetic variations, declination adjustments, and other factors that can influence compass accuracy, and ensure that you have the necessary knowledge and skills to navigate safely and confidently in the wilderness.

Embrace the journey, stay adaptable.

GPS Devices and Apps

Global Positioning System (GPS) devices and apps offer advanced navigation features, providing wilderness enthusiasts with real-time tracking, waypoint marking, and route planning capabilities. When selecting GPS devices and apps, consider the following factors:

GPS Devices:

Battery Life: Ensure the GPS device has an adequate battery life, considering the duration of your wilderness adventure and the availability of charging options.

Water Resistance: Look for GPS devices with water-resistant or waterproof designs to ensure functionality in various weather conditions.

Durability: opt for GPS devices with rugged and durable designs, capable of withstanding the rigors of wilderness exploration.

Display: Consider the device's display, ensuring it's readable in various lighting conditions, and offers a clear and intuitive interface.

Backup Power: Carry backup power sources, such as portable chargers or extra batteries, to ensure continuous operation in case of emergencies.

GPS Apps:

Compatibility: Ensure the GPS app is compatible with your mobile device and operating system, and that it offers offline map capabilities.

Battery Consumption: Monitor the app's battery consumption, as GPS usage can quickly drain your device's battery. Carry backup power sources, such as portable chargers, to ensure continuous operation.

Interface and Features: Evaluate the app's interface and features, ensuring they meet your navigation and wilderness exploration needs.

Offline Maps: Download offline maps before your adventure to ensure access to navigation data in areas without cellular coverage.

Reliability: Research the app's reliability, user reviews, and any known issues or limitations.

While GPS devices and apps provide valuable navigation tools, always carry a traditional compass and topographic map as a backup and for learning purposes. Familiarize yourself with the fundamentals of wilderness navigation, as over-reliance on electronic devices can lead to critical errors in judgment and decision-making.

Two-Way Radios and Satellite Phones

Effective communication is a crucial aspect of wilderness exploration, allowing you to stay connected with your group and access help in case of emergencies. Two-way radios and satellite phones enable communication in remote locations where cell phone coverage may be limited or non-existent. When selecting these communication tools, prioritize factors such as range, battery life, and ease of use. Familiarize yourself with emergency communication protocols and ensure you have a reliable means of contacting emergency services if needed.

Two-way Radios:

Two-way radios, also known as walkie-talkies, provide short-range, wireless communication between two or more individuals. Key factors to consider when selecting two-way radios include:

Range: Understand the radio's advertised range and consider factors that can affect transmission, such as terrain, obstacles, and weather conditions.

Battery Life: Check the battery life of the radio, and consider carrying extra batteries or rechargeable options to ensure continuous operation.

Ease of Use: opt for radios with user-friendly interfaces, clear audio quality, and straightforward controls to facilitate efficient communication.

Durability: Look for radios with rugged and durable designs, capable of withstanding the rigors of wilderness exploration.

Privacy Codes: Consider radios with privacy codes or squelch features, which can help reduce background noise and minimize interference from other users.

Satellite Phones:

Satellite phones provide long-range communication capabilities by connecting to orbiting satellites. Key factors to consider when selecting satellite phones include:

Coverage: Understand the satellite phone's coverage area, as some providers may have limited or no coverage in specific regions.

Battery Life: Check the battery life of the satellite phone, and consider carrying extra batteries or rechargeable options to ensure continuous operation.

Ease of Use: opt for satellite phones with user-friendly interfaces, clear audio quality, and straightforward controls to facilitate efficient communication.

Durability: Look for satellite phones with rugged and durable designs, capable of withstanding the rigors of wilderness exploration.

Cost: Consider the cost of satellite phone rentals or purchases, as well as the per-minute usage fees, which can be significantly higher than traditional cell phone plans.

Emergency Communication Protocols:

Familiarize yourself with emergency communication protocols and best practices, such as:

Establishing Check-In Points: Set up check-in points with your group, where you'll communicate your location, status, and any concerns.

Carrying a Distress Signal: Carry a distress signal, such as a whistle or flare, to attract attention in case of emergencies.

Memorizing Important Phone Numbers: Memorize important phone numbers, such as emergency services and personal contacts, in case your device is lost, stolen, or malfunctions.

Sharing Your Plans: Share your wilderness itinerary and contact information with a trusted friend or family member, so they can alert authorities if needed.

Using Appropriate Communication Devices: Choose the right communication tool for your wilderness adventure, considering factors such as range, battery life, and ease of use.

By carefully selecting and familiarizing yourself with two-way radios and satellite phones, you can ensure effective communication in remote locations and increase your safety and confidence during wilderness exploration. Following emergency communication protocols and having a reliable means of contacting emergency services will help you prepare for and manage unexpected situations in the wilderness

Personal Locator Beacons (PLBs) and Emergency Position Indicating Radio Beacons (EPIRBs)

Personal Locator Beacons (PLBs) and Emergency Position Indicating Radio Beacons (EPIRBs) are essential communication tools designed to send distress signals to search and rescue teams in the event of an emergency. These devices can be lifesaving in critical situations and should be considered an essential part of any prepping equipment kit.

Personal Locator Beacons (PLBs):

PLBs are compact, portable devices that emit a distress signal when activated, alerting search and rescue teams to your location. Key factors to consider when selecting PLBs include:

Size and Weight: opt for compact and lightweight PLBs that are easy to carry and stow in your backpack or survival kit.

Battery Life: Check the battery life of the PLB, ensuring it provides sufficient operation time in case of emergencies.

Activation Method: Familiarize yourself with the activation method, which typically involves deploying an antenna and pressing a button.

Integration with GPS: Look for PLBs with integrated GPS, as this can significantly reduce the time required to locate and rescue individuals in distress.

Waterproof and Floatation Capabilities: Prioritize PLBs with waterproof and floatation capabilities, ensuring operation in various weather conditions and environments.

Emergency Position Indicating Radio Beacons (EPIRBs):

EPIRBs are similar to PLBs but are designed for maritime use, transmitting a distress signal to the global Coast Guard rescue coordination centres. Key factors to consider when selecting EPIRBs include:

Mounting and Carrying: Determine whether the EPIRB will be mounted or carried, as this will influence the device's design, size, and weight.

Battery Life: Check the battery life of the EPIRB, ensuring it provides sufficient operation time in case of emergencies.

Integration with GPS: Look for EPIRBs with integrated GPS, as this can significantly reduce the time required to locate and rescue individuals in distress.

Waterproof and Floatation Capabilities: Prioritize EPIRBs with waterproof and floatation capabilities, ensuring operation in various maritime environments and conditions.

Registration and Cost: Ensure the EPIRB is registered with the appropriate authorities, and consider the cost of purchasing or renting the device.

Emergency Communication Best Practices:

Follow these emergency communication best practices when using PLBs and EPIRBs:

Activation: Activate the PLB or EPIRB only in life-threatening situations or when help is urgently needed.

Positioning: Ensure the device is positioned appropriately for optimal signal transmission, such as on a stable, elevated surface.

Notification: Notify emergency services and personal contacts of your situation, even if you have activated a PLB or EPIRB, as this can help expedite rescue efforts.

Deactivation: Deactivate the device once rescue is complete to avoid unnecessary searches and potential false alarms.

By incorporating PLBs or EPIRBs into your prepping equipment kit, you can enhance your safety and peace of mind during wilderness exploration and maritime adventures. Remember to adhere to emergency communication best practices and register EPIRBs with the appropriate authorities to ensure efficient and effective rescue operations in case of emergencies.

Additional Considerations for Your Navigation and Communication Toolkit

When building your navigation and communication toolkit, consider adding these additional components to enhance your wilderness experience and ensure safety during outdoor excursions:

Durable, Waterproof Cases: Invest in high-quality, waterproof cases that protect your navigation and communication devices from the elements, ensuring their continued functionality and longevity.

Extra Batteries, Chargers, or Solar Panels: Carry extra batteries, chargers, or portable solar panels to ensure continuous power during extended outdoor excursions and minimize the risk of device failure due to low battery levels.

Waterproof Notepads and Pencils: Bring waterproof notepads and pencils to record waypoints, bearings, and other essential navigation information, as well as to document observations, experiences, and memories.

Mirrors, Whistles, or Other Signalling Devices: Equip yourself with signalling devices, such as mirrors, whistles, or flare guns, to attract attention in case of emergency, making it easier for rescuers to locate and assist you.

Navigation Apps and Offline Maps: Utilize navigation apps and download offline maps on your smartphone for backup navigation purposes, providing an extra layer of redundancy and versatility in case primary navigation tools fail or are misplaced.

Spare Parts and Repair Kits: Carry spare parts, such as fuses, antennas, or small tools, and repair kits for your navigation and communication devices to address minor malfunctions or damage during outdoor adventures.

Learning Resources and Practice: Continuously expand your knowledge of navigation and communication techniques, tools, and best practices by engaging in learning resources, such as books, online courses, or workshops, and practicing your skills in various outdoor settings.

By incorporating these additional components and best practices into your navigation and communication toolkit, you can maximize your wilderness experience, enhance safety, and overcome potential challenges with confidence and preparedness.

Embrace the journey, stay adaptable

Chapter 4: Fire and Heat Production Essentials

Introduction

Fire and heat production are crucial for outdoor survival, providing warmth, cooking capabilities, and a means of signalling for help. This chapter will discuss various fire and heat production methods and tools to help you stay safe and comfortable during your wilderness adventures.

Fire Starters

Fire Starters: Essential Tools for Igniting Fires Quickly and Reliably

Fire starters are crucial tools for igniting fires quickly and reliably in various outdoor settings. They are compact, lightweight, and highly durable, making them ideal for inclusion in your prepping equipment kit. Consider the following fire starter options:

Ferrocerium Rods: Ferrocerium rods are compact, robust fire starters made of a ferrocerium alloy that produces sparks when scraped with a hard edge. They are weather-resistant, long-lasting, and can be easily attached to a keychain, multitool, or zipper pull for quick access.

Magnesium Fire Starters: Magnesium fire starters comprise a small magnesium block and a ferrocerium rod. To use, shave off thin flakes of magnesium, gather them into a small pile, and strike the ferrocerium rod to create sparks, which ignite the magnesium shavings. This method provides a dependable, waterproof fire-starting solution, even in wet or inclement conditions.

Flint and Steel Sets: Flint and steel sets consist of a piece of flint and a small, hardened steel striker. When struck together, they produce sparks, which can ignite tinder, kindling, or other combustible materials. These sets are time-tested, reliable fire-starting tools that are well-suited for outdoor enthusiasts and preppers.

Plasma Lighters: Plasma lighters use an electric arc to ignite fires, offering a windproof, waterproof, and highly dependable fire-starting solution. They are rechargeable, compact, and lightweight, making them an excellent addition to your prepping equipment kit.

Fire Pistons: Fire pistons are compact devices that use rapid compression to ignite a small piece of tinder, which can then be transferred to kindling or other fuel sources. They are easy to use, highly reliable, and can be used in wet or windy conditions.

When selecting a fire starter, consider factors such as dependability, ease of use, weight, size, and resistance to adverse weather conditions. By incorporating fire starters into your prepping equipment kit, you'll be better prepared to start fires in various outdoor environments, enhancing your ability to cook, stay warm, and signal for help if required.

Matches and Lighters

Matches and Lighters: Simple, Yet Effective Fire-starting Tools

Matches and lighters are simple, yet effective fire-starting tools that are indispensable for outdoor enthusiasts and preppers. These tools are compact, lightweight, and easy to use, making them an excellent addition to your prepping equipment kit. To ensure reliable performance under various weather conditions, consider opting for waterproof, windproof, or stormproof matches and lighters.

Waterproof Matches: Waterproof matches are treated with a water-resistant coating or wax that prevents moisture absorption, ensuring they remain functional even when wet. They are often sold in waterproof containers or matchboxes, which further protect the matches from moisture and the elements. Look for matches that produce a large spark and burn for an extended period to ensure the best results.

Windproof and Stormproof Matches: Windproof and stormproof matches are designed to withstand strong winds and adverse weather conditions, offering reliable ignition even in challenging outdoor environments. They typically feature a larger strike surface and burn for an extended period, allowing you to easily ignite tinder and kindling.

Lighters: Lighters are compact, portable fire-starting tools that offer quick and convenient ignition. Classic lighters, such as Bic or Zippo lighters, are inexpensive, readily available, and easy to use. However, they may not perform as well under adverse weather conditions. opt for waterproof, windproof, or stormproof lighters to ensure dependable performance in various outdoor settings.

Multi-tool Lighters: Multi-tool lighters, such as those that incorporate a bottle opener, scissors, or knife, can serve multiple purposes in a survival situation. These lighters are available in various designs, including rechargeable and disposable options.

Candle Lighters: Candle lighters are compact, portable lighters designed for lighting candles or other hard-to-reach areas. They often feature a long, flexible neck and a trigger-activated ignition mechanism, making them suitable for lighting fires in challenging environments.

When selecting matches or lighters, consider factors such as dependability, ease of use, weight, size, and resistance to adverse weather conditions. By incorporating these fire-starting tools into your prepping equipment kit, you'll be better prepared to start fires in various outdoor environments, enhancing your ability to cook, stay warm, and signal for help if required.

Tinder and Kindling

Tinder and kindling are indispensable fuel sources for starting and maintaining fires in various outdoor settings. Prepare a variety of tinder and kindling materials, such as dry leaves, grass, twigs, and small branches, before your outdoor excursions. In addition, consider carrying portable tinder alternatives for added convenience and versatility.

Natural Tinder and Kindling Materials

Dry Leaves and Grass: Gather dry leaves and grass from the ground or under the cover of trees and bushes. These materials ignite quickly and are ideal for starting fires in favourable weather conditions.

Twigs and Small Branches: Collect twigs and small branches, focusing on those with a diameter of less than a pencil. Break these branches into smaller pieces to facilitate ignition and ensure even burning.

Bark: Peel off dry bark from dead trees and branches. Many types of bark, such as birch bark, catch fire easily and burn for an extended period, making them excellent kindling materials.

Pine Needles and Cones: Pine needles and cones can be gathered and used as tinder or kindling. They ignite quickly and produce a long-lasting flame, perfect for starting fires in damp or humid environments.

Fatwood: Fatwood is the resin-rich heartwood of pine trees. It is highly flammable and can be easily split into small pieces or shavings to serve as tinder or kindling.

Portable Tinder Alternatives

Cotton Balls Soaked in Petroleum Jelly: Prepare portable tinder by soaking cotton balls in petroleum jelly. Store these tinder alternatives in a waterproof container, such as a small plastic bag or a waterproof matchbox. When needed, simply fluff the cotton ball to expose more surface area and ignite it with a spark or flame.

Dryer Lint: Collect dryer lint from your home's clothes dryer. Dryer lint is highly flammable and can be easily carried in a waterproof container. To use, fluff the lint to create more surface area and ignite it with a spark or flame.

Commercially Available Fire-starting Cubes: Purchase commercially available fire-starting cubes or tablets, which are designed to be portable, compact, and highly flammable. These products are often waterproof and can be ignited with a spark or flame, making them an excellent addition to your prepping equipment kit.

By preparing a variety of tinder and kindling materials and incorporating portable tinder alternatives into your prepping equipment kit, you can ensure reliable ignition and maintain burning in various outdoor environments. This will enhance your ability to cook, stay warm, and signal for help if required Fire Pits, Fire Rings, and Stoves

Fire pits, fire rings, and stoves provide a designated area for building and maintaining fires, helping to prevent accidental wildfires and ensuring more efficient fuel consumption. opt for lightweight, portable options that can be easily set up and dismantled in various environments.

Additional Considerations for Your Fire and Heat Production Kit

When building your fire and heat production kit, consider adding these additional components to enhance safety, versatility, and self-reliance during your outdoor excursions:

Fireproof Gloves or Mitts: Invest in high-quality fireproof gloves or mitts to protect your hands while handling hot materials, such as burning logs, coals, or metal fire accessories. These gloves are constructed from fire-resistant materials, such as aramid fibres or aluminized fabrics, and are available in various designs and sizes to suit your specific needs and preferences.

Fire Blankets or Extinguishers: Equip your fire and heat production kit with fire blankets or portable fire extinguishers to suppress accidental fires or control unpredictable burning conditions. Fire blankets are lightweight, compact, and easy to use, making them an excellent option for outdoor enthusiasts. Portable fire extinguishers, such as those designed for vehicle or marine use, can provide more substantial fire suppression capabilities in case of an emergency.

Multipurpose Tools: Incorporate multipurpose tools, such as a fire piston or bow drill, into your fire and heat production kit to enhance self-reliance and versatility in various outdoor environments. Fire pistons and bow drills are friction-based fire-starting tools that enable you to create fire without matches or lighters, providing an alternative ignition method in case your primary fire-starting tools fail or are lost.

Thermal Cookers or Insulated Pouches: Thermal cookers or insulated pouches are designed to retain heat and maintain the temperature of cooked food for extended periods. These devices can help reduce fuel consumption and cooking time, making them an excellent addition to your fire and heat production kit.

Heat Reflectors or Deflectors: Heat reflectors or deflectors can be used to direct and concentrate heat from your fire, improving cooking efficiency and reducing the amount of fuel required. These devices can be made from various materials, including aluminium foil, metal sheets, or heat-resistant fabrics.

Fire Rings or Portable Fire Pits: Fire rings or portable fire pits can help contain and manage your fire, reducing the risk of accidental fires and ensuring a safe and controlled burning environment. These devices are available in various materials, such as steel, cast iron, or titanium, and can be used in various outdoor settings, including campgrounds, backyards, or wilderness areas.

By incorporating these additional components and best practices into your fire and heat production kit, you can maximize your wilderness experience, enhance safety, and overcome potential challenges with confidence and preparedness.

Chapter 5: Water and Hygiene Equipment for Preppers

Introduction

Access to clean water and proper hygiene practices are essential for maintaining health and well-being during outdoor survival activities. This chapter will explore various water and hygiene equipment options to help you collect, purify, and manage water resources while minimizing the risk of illness and disease.

Water Collection and Filtration

Water Collection and Filtration: Crucial Techniques for Maintaining an Adequate Water Supply

Collecting and filtering water from natural sources is crucial for maintaining an adequate water supply during outdoor excursions. Various options are available to remove impurities, bacteria, and parasites from water sources, ensuring that the water you consume is safe and free from contaminants.

Portable Water Filters: Portable water filters, such as those using ceramic, carbon, or hollow-fibber membrane filtration technology, can effectively remove impurities, bacteria, and parasites from water sources. These filters are compact, lightweight, and easy to use, making them an excellent option for outdoor enthusiasts and preppers.

Gravity Filters: Gravity filters rely on the force of gravity to push water through a filtration system, removing impurities, bacteria, and parasites. These filters are available in various sizes and capacities, making them suitable for both individual and group use. They are often equipped with a reservoir, a filtration unit, and a collection container, providing a convenient and self-contained water filtration solution.

Life Straws: Life straws are personal, portable water filters designed for individual use. They feature a small, lightweight filtration unit that can be used to drink directly from a water source or in combination with a water bottle or hydration bladder. Life straws are an excellent option for lightweight backpacking, hiking, or camping, as they offer a simple, effective, and convenient water filtration solution.

Boiling: Boiling water is a simple and effective method for removing impurities, bacteria, and parasites. Bring water to a rolling boil for at least one minute (three minutes at higher elevations) to ensure that all contaminants have been eliminated. Allow the water to cool before consuming or storing it in a clean, food-grade container.

Chemical Treatment: Chemical treatments, such as chlorine or iodine tablets or drops, can be used to disinfect water and eliminate impurities, bacteria, and parasites. These treatments are compact, lightweight, and easy to use, making them an excellent option for outdoor enthusiasts and preppers. However, they may alter the taste and Odor of the water, and they may not be as effective at removing certain impurities as other filtration methods.

UV Light Treatment: UV light treatment devices, such as portable water purifiers or UV pens, can be used to eliminate impurities, bacteria, and parasites from water sources. These devices use ultraviolet light to destroy the DNA of microorganisms, rendering them harmless and safe for consumption. UV light treatment is a quick, effective, and chemical-free water purification method, but it may not be as effective at removing certain impurities as other filtration methods.

When collecting and filtering water from natural sources, it is essential to consider factors such as water availability, water quality, and water volume. By incorporating these water collection and filtration techniques into your prepping equipment kit, you can ensure a reliable and safe water supply during your outdoor excursions Water Purification

Water purification is an additional step to ensure water is safe for consumption. Boiling, chemicals, and UV light are common purification methods. opt for portable water purification tablets, drops, or UV light pens for added convenience and reliability.

Hygiene Essentials

Hygiene Essentials: Maintaining Proper Hygiene Practices in the Wilderness

Maintaining proper hygiene practices is crucial for preventing illness and disease during outdoor survival activities. Packing essential hygiene items, such as biodegradable soap, hand sanitizer, toothbrushes, toothpaste, toilet paper, and wipes, can help ensure that you remain clean and healthy throughout your wilderness experience.

Biodegradable Soap: Biodegradable soap is an environmentally friendly alternative to traditional soap, as it breaks down naturally and has minimal impact on the environment. Utilize biodegradable soap for washing hands, dishes, and clothing, ensuring that you minimize your environmental footprint while maintaining proper hygiene practices.

Hand Sanitizer: Hand sanitizer is a convenient and effective method for eliminating germs and bacteria on your hands. opt for alcohol-based hand sanitizers, which have been proven to be more effective at killing germs and bacteria than non-alcohol-based alternatives. Carry a small bottle of hand sanitizer in your pack, allowing for quick and easy sanitation throughout your wilderness excursion.

Toothbrushes and Toothpaste: Pack a compact toothbrush and travel-sized toothpaste to maintain oral hygiene during your outdoor adventure. Consider using a foldable or collapsible toothbrush to save space in your pack and minimize bulk.

Toilet Paper or Wipes: Pack a small supply of biodegradable toilet paper or wipes to use for personal hygiene during your outdoor excursion. If you opt for toilet paper, consider carrying a small, reusable container, such as a plastic bag or container, to store used toilet paper until it can be properly disposed of. If you prefer wipes, opt for biodegradable wipes, which break down naturally and have minimal impact on the environment.

Feminine Hygiene Products: For female adventurers, pack a sufficient supply of feminine hygiene products for your wilderness excursion. opt for reusable products, such as menstrual cups, to minimize waste and pack size.

Menstrual Supplies: For male adventurers, consider packing menstrual supplies, such as tampons or pads, for female companions during your wilderness adventure. This thoughtful gesture can help ensure that everyone in your group remains comfortable and prepared during their outdoor experience.

Nail Clippers and Tweezers: Pack a compact set of nail clippers and tweezers to maintain fingernail and toenail hygiene and remove unwanted splinters or debris from your skin.

When packing hygiene essentials, consider factors such as weight, size, and environmental impact. By incorporating these hygiene items into your prepping equipment kit, you can maintain proper hygiene practices during your outdoor excursions

Personal Hygiene

Personal hygiene practices, such as washing hands, brushing teeth, and cleaning dishes, help minimize the risk of illness and disease during outdoor survival activities. Opting for compact, lightweight hygiene products, such as collapsible buckets or sinks, can simplify these tasks and enhance your wilderness experience.

Collapsible Buckets or Sinks: Collapsible buckets or sinks are lightweight, portable, and easy to store, making them an excellent option for wilderness excursions. Utilize these collapsible containers for washing hands, dishes, and clothing, ensuring that you maintain proper hygiene practices without adding unnecessary weight or bulk to your pack.

Portable Water Filtration Systems: Portable water filtration systems, such as pump-style or gravity-fed filters, can provide clean, safe water for washing hands, dishes, and clothing. These systems are compact, lightweight, and easy to use, ensuring that you have access to clean water for personal hygiene tasks during your wilderness adventure.

Biodegradable Soap: Biodegradable soap, as previously mentioned, is an environmentally friendly alternative to traditional soap. Utilize biodegradable soap for washing hands, dishes, and clothing, ensuring that you minimize your environmental footprint while maintaining proper hygiene practices.

Hand Sanitizer: As previously mentioned, hand sanitizer is an effective method for eliminating germs and bacteria on your hands. Carry a small bottle of hand sanitizer in your pack, allowing for quick and easy sanitation throughout your wilderness excursion.

Compact Toothbrushes and Toothpaste: As previously mentioned, compact toothbrushes and travel-sized toothpaste are essential items for maintaining oral hygiene during outdoor adventures. opt for lightweight and space-saving designs to simplify packing and minimize pack weight.

Fast-Drying Towels: Fast-drying towels are lightweight, compact, and absorbent, making them an excellent option for wilderness excursions. Utilize these towels for drying hands, dishes, and clothing, ensuring that you maintain proper hygiene practices without adding unnecessary weight or bulk to your pack.

Compact Dish Racks or Drainers: Compact dish racks or drainers are designed to be lightweight and portable, making them ideal for wilderness excursions. Utilize these compact dish racks or drainers for drying dishes and cookware, ensuring that you maintain proper hygiene practices without adding unnecessary weight or bulk to your pack.

When selecting hygiene products for your wilderness adventure, consider factors such as weight, size, and environmental impact. By incorporating these compact and lightweight hygiene products into your prepping equipment kit, you can simplify personal hygiene practices

Additional Considerations

Additional Considerations for Your Water and Hygiene Equipment Kit

When building your water and hygiene equipment kit, consider incorporating these additional components to enhance convenience, cleanliness, and waste management during your wilderness excursions.

Water Bladders or Collapsible Water Containers: Water bladders or collapsible water containers are designed to be lightweight and portable, making them ideal for transporting and storing water during outdoor activities. These containers can be filled at natural water sources and connected to portable water filtration systems for on-the-go access to clean water.

Resealable Plastic Bags: Adequate waste management supplies, such as resealable plastic bags, are essential for disposing of used hygiene products and waste properly. Utilize resealable plastic bags for storing and transporting used hygiene products, trash, and recyclables, ensuring that you maintain a clean and sanitary wilderness environment.

Drying Lines and Clothespins: Drying lines, clothespins, or other drying equipment are crucial for maintaining cleanliness and drying wet items during extended outdoor excursions. Utilize drying lines and clothespins to hang wet clothing, towels, and other items, allowing them to air dry and reducing the risk of Mold and mildew growth.

Camp Sinks or Washbasins: Camp sinks or washbasins are lightweight, portable, and easy to store, making them an excellent option for wilderness excursions. Utilize these collapsible containers for washing hands, dishes, and clothing, ensuring that you maintain proper hygiene practices without adding unnecessary weight or bulk to your pack.

Personal Wet Wipes: Personal wet wipes are compact, lightweight, and disposable, making them an ideal option for quick and easy personal hygiene tasks during wilderness excursions. opt for biodegradable wet wipes to minimize environmental impact and ensure proper disposal.

Travel-Size Toiletries: Travel-size toiletries, such as shampoo, conditioner, and lotion, can be carried in a compact toiletry kit, allowing for easy transportation and storage during wilderness excursions. opt for biodegradable or eco-friendly alternatives to minimize environmental impact.

First Aid Kits: First aid kits are essential for addressing minor injuries, cuts, and scrapes during wilderness excursions. Ensure that your first aid kit includes items such as adhesive bandages, gauze pads, antiseptic wipes, tweezers, and pain relievers.

When selecting additional components for your water and hygiene equipment kit, consider factors such as weight, size, and environmental impact. By incorporating these additional considerations into your prepping equipment kit, you can enhance convenience, cleanliness, and waste management during your outdoor excursions

Chapter 6: Food and Nutrition Tools and Gadgets

Introduction

Proper nutrition is essential for maintaining energy levels and overall health during outdoor survival activities. This chapter will explore various food and nutrition tools and gadgets to help you collect, store, prepare, and cook meals during your wilderness adventures.

Food Collection and Preservation

Food Collection and Preservation: Strategies for Procuring and Preserving Nutrients During Wilderness Excursions

Collecting and preserving food from natural sources, such as hunting, fishing, and foraging, can provide essential nutrients and calories during outdoor excursions. Opting for portable, lightweight tools and food preservation methods can enhance your self-reliance and contribute to a more enjoyable and sustainable wilderness experience.

Hunting and Fishing Tools: Portable, lightweight hunting and fishing tools, such as fishing rods, traps, snares, and slingshots, can be carried in your pack, allowing you to procure food from natural sources during your wilderness excursion. Familiarize yourself with local hunting and fishing regulations, and obtain the necessary permits and licenses before embarking on your adventure.

Foraging Equipment: Foraging equipment, such as a small knife, field guide, and collection containers, can help you identify and collect wild edibles during your outdoor adventure. Familiarize yourself with local flora and fauna, and ensure that you only consume plants and mushrooms that are safe and edible.

Food Preservation Methods: Food preservation methods, such as dehydrated or freeze-dried food, mylar bags, and oxygen absorbers, can help preserve food collected from natural sources, ensuring that you have a reliable and sustainable food supply during your wilderness excursion.

Dehydrated or Freeze-Dried Food: Dehydrated or freeze-dried food is a convenient and lightweight option for carrying and preserving food during outdoor activities. These food products have a long shelf life and can be rehydrated with water, providing a quick and easy meal option during your wilderness adventure.

Mylar Bags and Oxygen Absorbers: Mylar bags and oxygen absorbers are effective food preservation methods for storing and preserving food collected from natural sources. Place dried food, such as fruits, vegetables, or meat, into a mylar bag, add an oxygen absorber, and seal the bag using a heat sealer or iron. This method creates an airtight and waterproof environment, ensuring that food remains fresh and edible for extended periods.

Smoking or Jerky Making: Smoking or jerky making is a traditional food preservation method that can be used to preserve meat, fish, and poultry during wilderness excursions. Utilize a portable, lightweight smoker or jerky maker to preserve meat, ensuring that you have a reliable and sustainable food supply during your outdoor adventure.

Canning or Pickling: Canning or pickling is a food preservation method that can be used to preserve fruits, vegetables, and meats during wilderness excursions. Utilize a portable, lightweight canning or pickling kit to preserve food, ensuring that you have a reliable and sustainable food supply during your outdoor adventure.

When selecting tools and methods for food collection and preservation, consider factors such as weight, size, and ease of use. By incorporating these strategies into your prepping equipment kit, you can enhance self-reliance, provide essential nutrients and calories, and contribute to a more enjoyable and safer wilderness experience.

Embrace the journey, stay adaptable

Food Storage

Food Storage: Techniques for Maintaining Freshness and Preventing Spoilage During Outdoor Excursions

Proper food storage is crucial for maintaining freshness and preventing spoilage during extended outdoor excursions. Opting for lightweight, portable food storage containers such as vacuum-sealed bags, airtight containers, or bear canisters can enhance your self-reliance and contribute to a safer and more enjoyable wilderness experience.

Vacuum-Sealed Bags: Vacuum-sealed bags are a lightweight and portable option for storing and preserving food during outdoor activities. These bags remove air and create an airtight seal, preventing moisture, bacteria, and Odors from affecting the food. Utilize vacuum-sealed bags to store dry goods, such as grains, nuts, and dried fruits, as well as cooked or raw meats, fish, and poultry.

Airtight Containers: Airtight containers are an excellent option for storing food during wilderness excursions. These containers prevent moisture, bacteria, and Odors from affecting the food, ensuring that it remains fresh and edible for an extended period. opt for lightweight and portable airtight containers made of durable materials, such as silicone or stainless steel, to store dry goods, cooked or raw meats, and other food items.

Bear Canisters: Bear canisters are compact, lightweight, and durable containers designed to prevent bears and other wildlife from accessing food and scented items during wilderness excursions. These canisters are typically made of hard plastic or aluminium and are equipped with airtight lids and secure latches. Utilize bear canisters to store food, cookware, and other scented items, ensuring that you maintain a safe and sanitary wilderness environment.

Food Coolers: Food coolers are an effective option for storing perishable food items during wilderness excursions. These coolers are designed to maintain a consistent temperature, preventing bacteria growth and spoilage. opt for lightweight and portable coolers with insulated walls and an airtight lid, ensuring that your perishable food items remain fresh and edible for an extended period.

Hanging Food Storage: Hanging food storage is an effective technique for preventing bears and other wildlife from accessing food during wilderness excursions. Utilize a lightweight and portable food storage bag or container, and attach it to a tree branch or other high and secure location, ensuring that your food remains safe and secure.

Food Hanging Hardware: Food hanging hardware, such as a carabiner, pulleys, or rope, can be used to securely hang food storage bags or containers from tree branches or other high and secure locations. opt for lightweight and portable hardware made of durable materials, ensuring that your food remains safe and secure during wilderness excursions.

Food Organization: Proper food organization is crucial for maintaining freshness and preventing spoilage during outdoor activities. Organize your food into categories, such as breakfast, lunch, dinner, and snacks, and store them in separate containers or compartments. Additionally, rotate your food storage regularly, consuming older items first to ensure that food remains fresh and edible.

When selecting food storage containers and techniques, consider factors such as weight, size, durability, and ease of use. By incorporating these strategies into your prepping equipment kit, you can maintain freshness, prevent spoilage, and contribute to a safer and more enjoyable wilderness experience.

Cooking Tools and Utensils

Cooking tools and utensils enable you to prepare hot meals and beverages during your outdoor survival activities. Opting for lightweight, compact options such as titanium pots, pans, cups, bowls, and utensils can enhance your self-reliance and contribute to a more enjoyable and sustainable wilderness experience.

Titanium Pots and Pans: Titanium pots and pans are an excellent option for cooking during wilderness excursions. These lightweight and durable cookware items are resistant to corrosion, scratches, and dents, ensuring that they can withstand the rigors of outdoor activities. Additionally, titanium has excellent heat conduction properties, allowing you to cook food evenly and efficiently.

Titanium Cups and Bowls: Titanium cups and bowls are compact, lightweight, and durable options for consuming hot meals and beverages during wilderness excursions. These items are typically designed with folding handles or collapsible designs, making them easy to store and transport.

Titanium Utensils: Titanium utensils, such as spoons, forks, and sporks, are lightweight, compact, and durable options for preparing and consuming meals during wilderness excursions. These items are typically designed with folding or collapsible handles, making them easy to store and transport.

Portable Stoves and Fuels: Portable stoves and fuels are essential for cooking during wilderness excursions. opt for lightweight and compact stoves that use readily available fuels, such as propane, butane, or wood. Additionally, ensure that your stove is equipped with safety features, such as flame regulators or wind shields, to ensure safe and efficient operation.

Multi-Tools: Multi-tools, such as a Swiss Army knife or Leatherman, are compact and versatile tools that can be used for a variety of tasks during wilderness excursions, including food preparation. These tools typically include features such as knives, can openers, scissors, and bottle openers, making them an essential addition to your cooking tools and utensils kit.

Camping Grills or Grill Pans: Camping grills or grill pans are compact, lightweight, and portable options for grilling during wilderness excursions. Utilize these grills or grill pans to cook meat, fish, or vegetables over an open flame, ensuring that you have a reliable and sustainable food supply during your outdoor adventure.

Folding or Collapsible Cutting Boards: Folding or collapsible cutting boards are lightweight, compact, and portable options for preparing food during wilderness excursions. Utilize these cutting boards to chop, dice, or slice food items, ensuring that you maintain proper food safety and hygiene practices during your outdoor adventure.

When selecting cooking tools and utensils, consider factors such as weight, size, durability, and versatility. By incorporating these strategies and equipment into your prepping equipment kit, you can prepare hot meals and beverages, maintain proper food safety and hygiene practices.

Food Preparation and Cooking Methods

Selecting appropriate food preparation and cooking methods can help conserve fuel, minimize equipment requirements, and maximize nutritional value during wilderness excursions. opt for versatile cooking methods such as boiling, simmering, frying, or baking using portable stoves, campfires, or integrated cooking systems.

Boiling or Simmering: Boiling or simmering is a versatile cooking method that can be used for preparing soups, stews, pasta, rice, and grains. Utilize a portable stove or campfire to bring water to a boil, and then add food items, allowing them to cook at a simmer. This method is efficient and can help conserve fuel, as it requires minimal heat input.

Frying: Frying is an effective cooking method for preparing meat, fish, or vegetables during wilderness excursions. Utilize a portable stove or campfire to heat oil or fat in a pan or frying basket, and then add food items, allowing them to cook until crispy and golden brown. This method can be used for preparing a variety of meals and can help enhance the flavour and texture of food items.

Baking: Baking is an effective cooking method for preparing bread, cakes, or other baked goods during wilderness excursions. Utilize a portable stove or campfire to heat a cast iron skillet or Dutch oven, and then add food items, allowing them to cook until golden brown and crispy. This method can be used for preparing a variety of meals and can help enhance the flavour and texture of food items.

Roasting or Grilling: Roasting or grilling is an effective cooking method for preparing meat, fish, or vegetables during wilderness excursions. Utilize a portable stove, campfire, or camping grill to cook food items over an open flame, ensuring that they are cooked evenly and thoroughly. This method can be used for preparing a variety of meals and can help enhance the flavour and texture of food items.

Insulated Cooking Systems: Insulated cooking systems, such as a thermal cooker or vacuum flask, can be used to cook food items using minimal heat input. Utilize a portable stove to bring food to a boil, and then transfer it to an insulated cooking system, allowing it to cook slowly and evenly. This method can help conserve fuel and minimize equipment requirements during wilderness excursions.

Dehydrated or Freeze-Dried Food: Dehydrated or freeze-dried food is a convenient and lightweight option for preparing hot meals during outdoor activities. Utilize a portable stove or campfire to rehydrate these food products, ensuring that you have a reliable and sustainable food supply during your wilderness adventure.

Food Preparation Techniques: Proper food preparation techniques are crucial for maintaining freshness and preventing spoilage during outdoor activities. Utilize techniques such as chopping, slicing, or dicing food items to ensure that they cook evenly and thoroughly. Additionally, consider using marinades or seasonings to enhance the flavour and texture of food items during wilderness excursions.

When selecting food preparation and cooking methods, consider factors such as fuel efficiency, equipment requirements, and nutritional value. By incorporating these strategies into your prepping equipment kit, you can conserve fuel, minimize equipment requirements, and maximize nutritional value during your outdoor excursions.

Additional Considerations

When building your food and nutrition tools and gadgets kit, consider including additional components such as:

Portable Spice Containers: Portable spice containers are compact, lightweight, and airtight containers that can be used to store and carry your favourite herbs and spices during wilderness excursions. Utilize these containers to enhance the flavour and enjoyment of meals, ensuring that you maintain a diverse and balanced diet during your outdoor adventure.

Multipurpose Tools: Multipurpose tools, such as a spork or multitool, can simplify food preparation and eating during wilderness excursions. opt for lightweight and compact tools that include features such as a spoon, fork, knife, can opener, bottle opener, or scissors, ensuring that you have a versatile and reliable tool for a variety of tasks.

Collapsible or Compact Measuring Cups and Spoons: Collapsible or compact measuring cups and spoons are compact, lightweight, and portable options for precise food preparation and portion control during wilderness excursions. Utilize these measuring cups and spoons to accurately measure and control the amount of food and ingredients used during wilderness excursions, ensuring that you maintain a healthy and balanced diet.

Food Thermometer: A food thermometer is an essential tool for ensuring that food items are cooked to the proper temperature during wilderness excursions. Utilize a portable and compact food thermometer to accurately measure the internal temperature of food items, ensuring that they are cooked thoroughly and safely.

Water Filter or Purifier: A water filter or purifier is an essential tool for ensuring that water is safe and potable during wilderness excursions. opt for lightweight and portable water filters or purifiers that can remove bacteria, viruses, and other contaminants from water sources, ensuring that you have a reliable and sustainable water supply during your outdoor adventure.

Portable Refrigeration or Cooling System: A portable refrigeration or cooling system is an effective tool for storing and preserving perishable food items during wilderness excursions. Utilize a lightweight and compact refrigeration or cooling system, such as a portable cooler or thermoelectric cooler, to maintain a consistent temperature, preventing bacteria growth and spoilage.

Emergency Food Rations: Emergency food rations, such as high-energy bars, trail mix, or military-style rations, are compact, lightweight, and calorie-dense options for maintaining energy and nutrition during wilderness excursions. Utilize these emergency food rations as a backup or supplemental food source during your outdoor adventure.

When selecting additional components for your food and nutrition tools and gadgets kit, consider factors such as weight, size, durability, and ease of use. By incorporating these additional components, you can enhance flavour, simplify food preparation

Chapter 7: Security and Protection Equipment

Introduction

Protecting yourself from potential hazards and threats is an essential aspect of outdoor survival. This chapter will explore various security and protection equipment options to help you stay safe and secure during your wilderness adventures.

Personal Protection

Personal protection equipment and strategies are crucial for deterring potential threats and providing peace of mind during outdoor activities. opt for personal protection equipment such as pepper spray, bear spray, or a personal alarm, and familiarize yourself with local regulations regarding the use and carry of these devices.

Pepper Spray or Bear Spray: Pepper spray or bear spray are effective personal protection tools for deterring potential threats during wilderness excursions. opt for lightweight and compact pepper spray or bear spray devices that can be easily carried and accessed during outdoor activities. Additionally, ensure that these devices are equipped with safety features, such as a flip-top or a locking mechanism, to prevent accidental discharge.

Personal Alarm: A personal alarm is a compact and lightweight personal protection tool that can be used to deter potential threats during wilderness excursions. Utilize a personal alarm to emit a loud, piercing sound that can be heard from a distance, ensuring that you have a reliable and effective tool for alerting others in case of an emergency.

Familiarization with Local Regulations: Familiarize yourself with local regulations regarding the use and carry of personal protection devices during wilderness excursions. Ensure that you are aware of any restrictions or requirements related to the use and carry of pepper spray, bear spray, or personal alarms during your outdoor adventure.

Safety Training and Education: Participate in safety training and education programs related to personal protection during wilderness excursions. Utilize resources such as wilderness survival courses, outdoor education programs, or local ranger stations to learn about effective personal protection strategies and techniques.

Preparation and Planning: Preparation and planning are crucial for ensuring a safe and enjoyable wilderness experience. Utilize maps, compasses, GPS devices, or other navigation tools to plan your route and identify potential hazards or threats during your outdoor adventure.

Buddy System: Consider utilizing the buddy system during wilderness excursions, ensuring that you have a reliable and trusted partner to accompany you during your outdoor adventure. Utilize the buddy system to share responsibilities, such as food preparation, navigation, or personal protection, and to provide mutual support and assistance during your wilderness experience.

Precautionary Measures: Utilize precautionary measures to minimize potential threats and hazards during wilderness excursions. opt for brightly coloured or reflective clothing and gear, ensuring that you are visible and identifiable during outdoor activities. Additionally, consider using insect repellent, sunscreen, or other protective measures to minimize potential hazards during wilderness excursions.

When selecting personal protection equipment and strategies, consider factors such as weight, size, durability, and ease of use. By incorporating these personal protection equipment and strategies into your prepping equipment kit, you can deter potential threats, provide peace of mind, and contribute to a safer and more enjoyable wilderness experience.

Embrace the journey.

Wildlife Protection

Protecting yourself from wildlife encounters is crucial for maintaining safety during outdoor excursions. opt for portable, lightweight wildlife protection equipment, such as bear spray, horns, or electric fences, and learn about effective wildlife protection strategies and techniques.

Bear Spray and Horns: Bear spray and horns are effective wildlife protection tools for deterring potential threats during wilderness excursions. opt for lightweight and compact bear spray or horn devices that can be easily carried and accessed during outdoor activities. Additionally, ensure that these devices are equipped with safety features, such as a flip-top or a locking mechanism, to prevent accidental discharge.

Electric Fences: Electric fences are portable and lightweight wildlife protection tools that can be used to deter potential threats during wilderness excursions. Utilize electric fences to create a barrier around your campsite or food storage area, ensuring that you have a reliable and effective tool for protecting yourself from wildlife encounters.

Familiarization with Wildlife Protection Strategies and Techniques: Participate in wildlife protection training and education programs related to wildlife encounters during wilderness excursions. Utilize resources such as wilderness survival courses, outdoor education programs, or local ranger stations to learn about effective wildlife protection strategies and techniques.

Food Storage: Proper food storage is crucial for preventing wildlife encounters during wilderness excursions. Utilize bear-resistant containers or hang food bags from trees, ensuring that food items are stored safely and securely during your outdoor adventure.

Wildlife Awareness: Maintain a high level of wildlife awareness during wilderness excursions. Utilize resources such as maps, wildlife guides, or local ranger stations to learn about potential wildlife hazards or threats during your outdoor adventure.

Respect for Wildlife: Respect wildlife during wilderness excursions, ensuring that you maintain a safe and respectful distance from wildlife animals. Avoid approaching, feeding, or disturbing wildlife animals, ensuring that you maintain a safe and ethical relationship with wildlife during your outdoor adventure.

Insect and Pest Protection

Preventing insect and pest bites is essential for maintaining health and comfort during outdoor activities. Consider options such as insect repellent, permethrin-treated clothing, and mosquito nets to protect yourself from insect and pest bites.

Insect Repellent: Insect repellent is an effective tool for preventing insect and pest bites during wilderness excursions. opt for lightweight and compact insect repellent devices, such as sprays, lotions, or wipes, that can be easily carried and applied during outdoor activities.

Permethrin-Treated Clothing: Permethrin-treated clothing is an effective tool for preventing insect and pest bites during wilderness excursions. Utilize permethrin-treated clothing and gear, such as pants, shirts, socks, or hats, to protect yourself from insect and pest bites during your outdoor adventure.

Mosquito Nets: Mosquito nets are an effective tool for preventing insect and pest bites during wilderness excursions. Utilize mosquito nets to protect yourself from insect and pest bites while sleeping or resting, ensuring that you maintain a comfortable and insect-free environment during your outdoor adventure.

Familiarization with Insect and Pest Protection Strategies and Techniques: Participate in insect and pest protection training and education programs related to insect and pest protection during wilderness excursions. Utilize resources such as wilderness survival courses, outdoor education programs, or local ranger stations to learn about effective insect and pest protection strategies and techniques.

When selecting wildlife and insect protection equipment and strategies, consider factors such as weight, size, durability, and ease of use. By incorporating these wildlife and insect protection equipment and strategies into your prepping equipment kit, you can protect yourself from wildlife encounters, prevent insect and pest bites.

Chapter 8: First Aid and Medical Supplies for Preppers

Introduction

First aid and medical supplies are essential components of any outdoor survival kit. They enable you to address minor injuries, illnesses, or emergencies promptly and effectively.

Basic First Aid Kits

A basic first aid kit is an essential tool for providing medical assistance during outdoor activities. opt for compact, lightweight first aid kits that can be easily carried and accessed during outdoor activities and ensure that they include essential items such as adhesive bandages, gauze pads, antiseptic wipes, tweezers, and medical tape.

Adhesive Bandages: Adhesive bandages are an essential tool for providing medical assistance during outdoor activities. Utilize adhesive bandages to cover minor wounds, cuts, or scrapes, ensuring that they are protected from dirt, debris, and infection.

Gauze Pads: Gauze pads are an essential tool for providing medical assistance during outdoor activities. Utilize gauze pads to absorb blood, control bleeding, or protect larger wounds, ensuring that they are properly cleaned, dressed, and cared for during your outdoor adventure.

Antiseptic Wipes: Antiseptic wipes are an essential tool for providing medical assistance during outdoor activities. Utilize antiseptic wipes to clean and disinfect wounds, cuts, or scrapes, ensuring that they are free from dirt, debris, and bacteria that can cause infection.

Tweezers: Tweezers are an essential tool for providing medical assistance during outdoor activities. Utilize tweezers to remove splinters, ticks, or other foreign objects from wounds, cuts, or scrapes, ensuring that they are properly cleaned, dressed, and cared for during your outdoor adventure.

Medical Tape: Medical tape is an essential tool for providing medical assistance during outdoor activities. Utilize medical tape to secure bandages, dressings, or other medical supplies, ensuring that they remain in place and provide proper protection and support.

Additional First Aid Items: In addition to essential first aid items, consider including additional items such as pain relievers, antihistamines, or other over-the-counter medications, as well as emergency blankets, whistles, or other rescue signals in your first aid kit.

Familiarization with First Aid Strategies and Techniques: Participate in first aid training and education programs related to providing medical assistance during wilderness excursions. Utilize resources such as wilderness survival courses, outdoor education programs, or local ranger stations to learn about effective first aid strategies and techniques.

When selecting a basic first aid kit, consider factors such as weight, size, durability, and ease of use. By incorporating these first aid equipment and strategies into your prepping equipment kit, you can provide medical assistance, prevent infection.

Advanced First Aid Kits

An advanced first aid kit is designed for more serious injuries or emergencies, requiring specialized training and knowledge. opt for compact, lightweight advanced first aid kits that can be easily carried and accessed during outdoor activities and ensure that they include additional items such as trauma shears, splints, a tourniquet, airway management tools, and haemostatic agents.

Trauma Shears: Trauma shears are an essential tool for providing specialized medical assistance during outdoor activities. Utilize trauma shears to quickly and safely cut through clothing, bandages, or other materials, ensuring that you can access wounds, cuts, or scrapes during your outdoor adventure.

Splints: Splints are an essential tool for providing specialized medical assistance during outdoor activities. Utilize splints to immobilize injured limbs, joints, or bones, ensuring that they are protected from further damage or injury during your outdoor adventure.

Tourniquet: A tourniquet is an essential tool for providing specialized medical assistance during outdoor activities. Utilize a tourniquet to control severe bleeding, ensuring that you can provide lifesaving medical assistance during your outdoor adventure.

Airway Management Tools: Airway management tools are essential for providing specialized medical assistance during outdoor activities. opt for compact, lightweight airway management tools, such as oral or nasal airways, bag-valve masks, or portable oxygen devices, that can be easily carried and accessed during outdoor activities.

Haemostatic Agents: Haemostatic agents are essential for providing specialized medical assistance during outdoor activities. Utilize haemostatic agents, such as gauze pads or powders, to control severe bleeding, ensuring that you can provide lifesaving medical assistance during your outdoor adventure.

Specialized Training and Education: Participate in advanced first aid training and education programs related to providing specialized medical assistance during wilderness excursions. Utilize resources such as wilderness survival courses, outdoor education programs, or local ranger stations to learn about effective advanced first aid strategies and techniques.

Incorporation of Basic First Aid Strategies and Techniques: In addition to specialized first aid items, ensure that your advanced first aid kit includes essential items such as adhesive bandages, gauze pads, antiseptic wipes, tweezers, and medical tape. By incorporating both basic and advanced first aid strategies and techniques, you can provide comprehensive medical assistance during your outdoor adventure.

When selecting an advanced first aid kit, consider factors such as weight, size, durability, and ease of use. By incorporating these advanced first aid equipment and strategies into your prepping equipment kit, you can provide specialized medical assistance, control bleeding, manage airways.

Personal Medications

If you require prescription medications, it is crucial to ensure that you have an adequate supply for the duration of your outdoor excursion. Properly managing personal medications can contribute to a safer and more enjoyable wilderness experience.

Adequate Supply: Ensure that you have an adequate supply of personal medications for the duration of your outdoor excursion. Consult with your healthcare provider to determine the appropriate dosage and duration of your medication, and plan accordingly.

Original Containers: Carry personal medications in their original containers, which can help prevent confusion or errors during administration. Original containers also provide important information, such as dosage instructions, expiration dates, and pharmacy contact information.

Copy of Prescription and Doctor's Note: Carry a copy of your prescription and a doctor's note, if necessary, to help verify the legitimacy of your medications. This can be particularly important if you need to seek medical assistance during your outdoor adventure.

Proper Storage: Properly store personal medications during outdoor activities to ensure their stability and effectiveness. opt for containers that are waterproof, airtight, and light-resistant, and avoid storing medications in extreme temperatures or direct sunlight.

Emergency Contact Information: Carry emergency contact information, such as the phone number and address of your healthcare provider, pharmacy, or emergency contact, to help facilitate medical assistance during your outdoor adventure.

Familiarization with Medication Management Strategies and Techniques: Participate in medication management training and education programs related to managing personal medications during wilderness excursions. Utilize resources such as wilderness survival courses, outdoor education programs, or local ranger stations to learn about effective medication management strategies and techniques.

Disposal of Expired or Unused Medications: Properly dispose of expired or unused medications during or after your outdoor adventure. opt for environmentally friendly disposal methods, such as returning unused medications to a pharmacy or utilizing a medication disposal program, to help reduce environmental impact and promote sustainability.

When managing personal medications during outdoor activities, consider factors such as proper storage, adequate supply, and emergency contact information. By incorporating these medication management strategies and techniques into your prepping equipment kit, you can ensure the stability, effectiveness, and safety of your personal medications during your wilderness experience.

Embrace the journey.

Over-the-Counter Medications

Over-the-counter (OTC) medications, such as pain relievers, allergy pills, and anti-diarrheal tablets, can significantly enhance your outdoor experience by alleviating symptoms of minor ailments. By properly managing OTC medications, you can ensure a more comfortable and enjoyable wilderness adventure.

Selection of OTC Medications: Select a variety of OTC medications, tailored to the specific ailments or symptoms you may encounter during your outdoor excursion. opt for medications that are lightweight, compact, and easy to use. Some essential OTC medications include:

Pain relievers (acetaminophen, ibuprofen, or aspirin) for managing pain, fever, or inflammation

Allergy pills (antihistamines) for managing allergic reactions or itching

Anti-diarrheal tablets (loperamide) for managing diarrhoea or gastrointestinal discomfort

Antacids for managing indigestion, heartburn, or acid reflux

Topical creams or ointments for managing insect bites, rashes, or skin irritations

Proper Storage: Properly store OTC medications during outdoor activities to ensure their stability and effectiveness. opt for waterproof, airtight, and light-resistant containers, and avoid storing medications in extreme temperatures or direct sunlight. Clearly label each medication container with its name, dosage, and expiration date.

Dosage Instructions: Carefully follow dosage instructions for OTC medications, ensuring that you administer the appropriate dosage for your age, weight, and health status. Consult with a healthcare provider or pharmacist if you are unsure about the appropriate dosage or duration of OTC medication use.

Emergency Contact Information: Carry emergency contact information, such as the phone number and address of your healthcare provider, pharmacy, or emergency contact, to help facilitate medical assistance during your outdoor adventure.

Familiarization with Medication Management Strategies and Techniques: Participate in medication management training and education programs related to managing OTC medications during wilderness excursions. Utilize resources such as wilderness survival courses, outdoor education programs, or local ranger stations to learn about effective medication management strategies and techniques, such as:

Identifying and managing potential side effects or drug interactions

Administering medications using the correct techniques and equipment

Developing a medication schedule or routine to ensure proper dosage and timing

Monitoring and documenting medication use and response

Disposal of Expired or Unused Medications: Properly dispose of expired or unused medications during or after your outdoor adventure. opt for environmentally friendly disposal methods, such as returning unused medications to a pharmacy or utilizing a medication disposal program, to help reduce environmental impact and promote sustainability.

Emergency Medical Reference Guides

Carry Emergency Medical Reference Guides: Essential Equipment for Making Informed Decisions Regarding First Aid and Medical Treatments During Outdoor Excursions

Carrying emergency medical reference guides, such as a first aid manual or a wilderness first aid app, is an essential aspect of prepping for outdoor activities. These guides can significantly enhance your ability to make informed decisions regarding first aid and medical treatments during outdoor excursions.

Selection of Emergency Medical Reference Guides: Select emergency medical reference guides that are specifically designed for wilderness or outdoor settings. opt for guides that are comprehensive, easy to understand, and include illustrations or diagrams to help clarify concepts. First aid manuals, wilderness first aid apps, or emergency medical guides are some examples.

Familiarization with Guide Content: Familiarize yourself with the content of your selected emergency medical reference guide before embarking on your outdoor excursion. Review the guide's table of contents, index, and key concepts to ensure that you can quickly locate and utilize the information you need during an emergency.

Practical Application: Practice using your emergency medical reference guide in simulated emergency scenarios to ensure that you can effectively apply the information in real-life situations. This can help you build confidence in your ability to provide first aid and medical treatments during outdoor excursions.

Up-to-Date Information: Ensure that your emergency medical reference guide is up-to-date and includes the most recent information regarding first aid and medical treatments. Regularly review and update your guide as necessary to maintain its accuracy and relevance.

Accessibility: Carry your emergency medical reference guide in a location that is easily accessible during outdoor activities. opt for a waterproof or durable case to protect the guide from damage or exposure to the elements.

Integration with First Aid Kits: Integrate your emergency medical reference guide with your first aid kit to ensure that you have all the necessary tools and resources for providing first aid and medical treatments during outdoor excursions.

When prepping for your outdoor adventure, carefully consider the selection, familiarization, practical application, and accessibility of your emergency medical reference guides. Additional Considerations

When building your first aid and medical supplies kit, consider additional components such as:

A personal medical history form, including chronic conditions, allergies, and contact information for healthcare providers

Additional protective equipment, such as gloves or a face mask, to minimize the risk of infection during first aid procedures

A first aid training course or certification to ensure you have the knowledge and skills required to effectively administer first aid during outdoor activities.

Chapter 9: Power and Lighting Solutions for Outdoor Survival Living

Introduction

Power and lighting solutions are essential for maintaining functionality and safety during outdoor survival activities. This chapter will explore various power and lighting options to help you stay powered and illuminated during your wilderness adventures.

Portable Power Banks and Solar Chargers

Portable power banks and solar chargers are essential prepping equipment, enabling you to recharge devices, such as smartphones, GPS devices, or radios, during outdoor activities. opt for lightweight, compact options with multiple USB ports and fast charging capabilities to ensure that you can maintain communication and navigation devices during your adventure.

Selection of Portable Power Banks: Select portable power banks with high capacities, multiple USB ports, and fast charging capabilities. opt for power banks with high milliampere-hour (Mah) ratings, which can provide extended power for multiple devices. Additionally, consider power banks with built-in flashlights, compartments for storing cables, or other additional features that can enhance their functionality during outdoor activities.

Selection of Solar Chargers: Select solar chargers that are compact, lightweight, and durable. opt for chargers that can be easily attached to backpacks, tents, or other outdoor gear, allowing you to harness the power of the sun while on the move. Additionally, consider chargers with built-in batteries, USB ports, or other features that can enhance their functionality during outdoor activities.

Charging and Maintenance: Properly charge and maintain your portable power banks and solar chargers to ensure their longevity and effectiveness during outdoor activities. Regularly charge your power banks before embarking on your excursion, and avoid exposing them to extreme temperatures or direct sunlight. Additionally, clean your solar chargers with a soft, dry cloth to remove dirt, debris, or other contaminants that can affect their performance.

Integration with Other Devices: Integrate your portable power banks and solar chargers with other devices, such as smartphones, GPS devices, or radios, to ensure that you can maintain communication and navigation capabilities during your adventure. Ensure that your devices are compatible with your power banks and solar chargers, and opt for cables or adapters that can facilitate charging and power transfer.

Testing and Familiarization: Test and familiarize yourself with your portable power banks and solar chargers before embarking on your outdoor excursion. Understand their charging capabilities, charging times, and other key features to ensure that you can effectively utilize them during your adventure.

When prepping for your outdoor adventure, carefully consider the selection, charging, maintenance, integration, and testing of your portable power banks and solar chargers. Rechargeable Batteries and Battery Chargers

Rechargeable batteries and battery chargers can help reduce waste and save money during outdoor excursions. Consider options such as AA, AAA, or CR123A rechargeable batteries and portable chargers for your devices.

Dynamo or Crank-Powered Devices

Dynamo or crank-powered devices offer an alternative, eco-friendly method of generating power during outdoor activities. These devices use a hand crank or dynamo mechanism to convert mechanical energy into electrical energy, providing a reliable power source for various applications. opt for devices such as flashlights, radios, or phone chargers that can be powered by a hand crank or dynamo mechanism, ensuring that you have access to essential communication, lighting, or navigation tools during your adventure.

Selection of Dynamo Devices: Select dynamo devices that are compact, lightweight, and durable, and opt for devices that offer multiple functionalities. For instance, consider a flashlight with a built-in radio, phone charger, or other features that can enhance its versatility during outdoor activities.

Ergonomics and Design: Consider the ergonomics and design of your dynamo devices, ensuring that they are easy to grip, operate, and transport during outdoor activities. opt for devices with comfortable hand grips, sturdy construction, and integrated storage compartments for cables or other accessories.

Power Generation and Efficiency: Evaluate the power generation and efficiency of your dynamo devices, ensuring that they can provide sufficient power for your specific needs. opt for devices with high wattage ratings, fast charging capabilities, or other features that can enhance their power generation and efficiency during outdoor activities.

Integration with Other Devices: Integrate your dynamo devices with other devices, such as smartphones, GPS devices, or radios, to ensure that you can maintain communication and navigation capabilities during your adventure. Ensure that your devices are compatible with your dynamo devices, and opt for cables or adapters that can facilitate charging and power transfer.

Testing and Familiarization: Test and familiarize yourself with your dynamo devices before embarking on your outdoor excursion. Understand their power generation capabilities, charging times, and other key features to ensure that you can effectively utilize them during your adventure.

When prepping for your outdoor adventure, carefully consider the selection, ergonomics, power generation, integration, and testing of your dynamo or crank-powered devices. By incorporating these devices into your prepping equipment kit, you can enjoy an eco-friendly, reliable power source

Lighting Solutions

Lighting solutions are crucial for maintaining visibility during nighttime activities. opt for lightweight, compact options with long-lasting batteries, adjustable brightness settings, and durable construction, ensuring that you have access to reliable lighting tools during your adventure.

Selection of Lighting Solutions: Select lighting solutions that cater to your specific needs and preferences, such as headlamps, flashlights, or lanterns. opt for devices that offer adjustable brightness settings, multiple lighting modes, or other features that can enhance their functionality during outdoor activities.

Battery Life and Durability: Evaluate the battery life and durability of your lighting solutions, opting for devices with long-lasting batteries, low power consumption, or other features that can extend their runtime during outdoor activities. Consider investing in rechargeable batteries or solar-powered options to reduce battery waste and promote sustainability.

Weight and Portability: Consider the weight and portability of your lighting solutions, opting for lightweight, compact devices that are easy to transport during outdoor activities. opt for devices with integrated storage compartments, belt clips, or other features that can facilitate their transportation during your adventure.

Integration with Other Devices: Integrate your lighting solutions with other devices, such as smartphones, GPS devices, or radios, to ensure that you can maintain communication and navigation capabilities during your adventure. opt for devices with built-in USB ports, wireless charging capabilities, or other features that can facilitate their integration with other devices.

Testing and Familiarization: Test and familiarize yourself with your lighting solutions before embarking on your outdoor excursion. Understand their brightness settings, runtime, and other key features to ensure that you can effectively utilize them during your adventure.

Additional Considerations

When building your power and lighting solutions kit, consider additional components such as a portable, multi-function power station, LED light strips or lanterns, and solar-powered security or safety lights. These devices can significantly enhance your ability to power and illuminate your outdoor activities, ensuring that you have access to essential communication, navigation, and safety tools during your adventure.

Portable, Multi-Function Power Stations: opt for a portable, multi-function power station to power larger devices, such as laptops or CPAP machines, during extended outdoor excursions. These devices typically offer high milliampere-hour (Mah) ratings, multiple USB ports, and various output options, such as AC or DC outlets. When selecting a portable power station, consider its weight, size, and runtime, ensuring that it can meet your power needs while remaining portable and easy to transport.

LED Light Strips or Lanterns: Consider LED light strips or lanterns for area lighting during camping or basecamp activities. These devices offer bright, energy-efficient illumination, and can significantly enhance visibility during nighttime activities. opt for lightweight, compact options with adjustable brightness settings, multiple lighting modes, or other features that can enhance their functionality during outdoor activities.

Solar-Powered Security or Safety Lights: Invest in solar-powered security or safety lights to deter wildlife or provide illumination around your campsite. Solar-powered lights offer an eco-friendly, sustainable lighting solution, and can help ensure your safety and security during nighttime activities. opt for devices with motion sensors, adjustable brightness settings, or other features that can enhance their functionality during outdoor activities.

Integration of Power and Lighting Solutions: Integrate your power and lighting solutions with other devices, such as smartphones, GPS devices, or radios, to ensure that you can maintain communication, navigation, and safety capabilities during your adventure. opt for devices with built-in USB ports, wireless charging capabilities, or other features that can facilitate their integration with other devices.

Testing and Familiarization: Test and familiarize yourself with your power and lighting solutions before embarking on your outdoor excursion. Understand their power generation capabilities, charging times, brightness settings, and other key features to ensure that you can effectively utilize them during your adventure.

When prepping for your outdoor adventure, carefully consider the selection, integration, and testing of your power and lighting solutions. By incorporating these devices into your prepping equipment kit, you can enhance your ability to power and illuminate your outdoor activities.

Chapter 10: Preparing for Special Considerations and Eventualities

Introduction

Outdoor survival activities may present unique challenges or eventualities that require specialized equipment or strategies. This chapter will explore various special considerations and eventualities to help you prepare for a wider range of scenarios during your wilderness adventures.

Extreme Weather Conditions

Extreme weather conditions, such as cold temperatures, high winds, or heavy rain, can significantly impact your outdoor experience. opt for specialized equipment, such as waterproof clothing, insulated sleeping bags, or four-season tents, to protect yourself from the elements and maintain safety and comfort during challenging outdoor activities.

Waterproof Clothing: Invest in high-quality, waterproof clothing, such as rain jackets, pants, or boots, to protect yourself from heavy rain or wet snow. opt for breathable, lightweight materials that can prevent overheating, and consider features such as adjustable cuffs, waterproof zippers, or pit zips that can enhance their functionality during outdoor activities.

Insulated Sleeping Bags: Select insulated sleeping bags that cater to your specific temperature needs and conditions, such as down-filled or synthetic bags. opt for bags with adjustable hoods, draft collars, or other features that can enhance their insulation capabilities, and consider their weight, size, and compressibility, ensuring that they are easy to transport during outdoor activities.

Four-Season Tents: opt for four-season tents that are specifically designed for extreme weather conditions, offering enhanced durability, stability, and insulation. Consider features such as double-walled construction, waterproof materials, or adjustable vents that can enhance their functionality during outdoor activities.

Additional Preparations for Extreme Weather Conditions: In addition to specialized equipment, consider additional preparations for extreme weather conditions, such as:

Building snow shelters or windbreaks to protect yourself from harsh elements

Utilizing insulation materials, such as foam pads or reflective blankets, to enhance your warmth and comfort

Implementing proper hydration and nutrition strategies to maintain your energy levels and overall well-being during extreme weather conditions

Testing and Familiarization: Test and familiarize yourself with your extreme weather equipment before embarking on your outdoor excursion. Understand their insulation capabilities, waterproofing, and other key features to ensure that you can effectively utilize them during your adventure.

When prepping for your outdoor adventure, carefully consider the selection, functionality, and testing of your extreme weather equipment. By incorporating these devices into your prepping equipment kit, you can maintain safety, comfort.

Navigation in Challenging Terrain

Navigating challenging terrain, such as dense forests, steep slopes, or swamps, can present unique challenges during outdoor excursions. opt for specialized equipment, such as trekking poles, climbing gear, or specialized maps, to help you overcome obstacles and maintain safety during challenging outdoor activities.

Trekking Poles: Invest in high-quality trekking poles to provide additional stability and balance during challenging terrain. opt for adjustable, lightweight poles that can be easily transported during outdoor activities, and consider features such as ergonomic handles, shock-absorbing mechanisms, or mud baskets that can enhance their functionality during outdoor activities.

Climbing Gear: Select climbing gear that caters to your specific needs and conditions, such as harnesses, carabiners, or ropes. opt for gear that is lightweight, durable, and easy to use, and consider features such as adjustable buckles, locking mechanisms, or other features that can enhance their functionality during outdoor activities.

Specialized Maps: Utilize specialized maps, such as topographic maps, aerial photographs, or satellite imagery, to help you navigate challenging terrain. opt for maps that offer detailed information about the terrain, such as elevation contours, vegetation, or waterways, and consider features such as grid systems, scale indicators, or other features that can enhance their functionality during outdoor activities.

Additional Preparations for Challenging Terrain: In addition to specialized equipment, consider additional preparations for challenging terrain, such as:

Researching and studying the area before embarking on your excursion

Implementing proper safety measures, such as using safety ropes, harnesses, or other protective gear

Utilizing navigation tools, such as compasses, GPS devices, or smartphone apps, to help you maintain your bearings and avoid getting lost

Testing and Familiarization: Test and familiarize yourself with your challenging terrain equipment before embarking on your outdoor excursion. Understand their functionality, adjustability, and other key features to ensure that you can effectively utilize them during your adventure.

When prepping for your outdoor adventure, carefully consider the selection, functionality, and testing of your challenging terrain equipment. By incorporating these devices into your prepping equipment kit, you can overcome obstacles, maintain safety Water Crossings and Swimming

Water crossings and swimming can be hazardous during outdoor activities. opt for specialized equipment, such as personal flotation devices, water shoes, or dry bags, to help you navigate water safely.

Traveling with Children or Pets

Traveling with children or pets during outdoor activities requires additional considerations and equipment. opt for lightweight, portable items, such as collapsible water bowls, pet carriers, or child-carrying packs, to accommodate their needs during your wilderness adventures and ensure a safe, comfortable, and enjoyable experience for the whole family.

Collapsible Water Bowls: Invest in collapsible water bowls to provide your pets or children with access to fresh water during outdoor activities. opt for bowls that are lightweight, durable, and easy to clean, and consider features such as adjustable stands, carabiners, or other accessories that can enhance their functionality during outdoor activities.

Pet Carriers or Packs: Select pet carriers or packs that cater to your specific pet's size, weight, and needs. opt for carriers or packs that are lightweight, durable, and easy to transport, and consider features such as ventilation systems, adjustable straps, or pockets that can enhance their functionality during outdoor activities.

Child-Carrying Packs: opt for child-carrying packs that provide a comfortable, safe, and secure carrying solution for your child during outdoor activities. Consider features such as adjustable straps, ventilation systems, or pockets that can enhance their functionality, and ensure that they meet safety standards and regulations for outdoor activities.

Additional Preparations for Traveling with Children or Pets: In addition to specialized equipment, consider additional preparations for traveling with children or pets, such as:

Researching and studying the area before embarking on your excursion to ensure it is safe and suitable for children or pets

Implementing proper safety measures, such as using safety harnesses, leashes, or other protective gear

Providing ample rest, food, and water breaks during outdoor activities

Testing and Familiarization: Test and familiarize yourself with your traveling equipment before embarking on your outdoor excursion. Understand their functionality, adjustability, and other key features to ensure that you can effectively utilize them during your adventure and provide a safe, comfortable, and enjoyable experience for the whole family.

When prepping for your outdoor adventure with children or pets, carefully consider the selection, functionality, and testing of your travel equipment. By incorporating these devices into your prepping equipment kit, you can accommodate their needs, maintain safety and comfort, and contribute to a more rewarding wilderness experience for the whole family.

Additional Considerations

Addressing Unique Scenarios During Outdoor Activities

When preparing for outdoor activities, it is crucial to consider special considerations and eventualities, such as allergies, respiratory conditions, communication with emergency services, or long-term wilderness survival situations. opt for additional components, such as specialized first aid kits, satellite messengers, or portable water filters, to address these unique scenarios and ensure a safe, comfortable, and enjoyable experience during your wilderness adventures.

Specialized First Aid Kits or Medical Supplies: Invest in specialized first aid kits or medical supplies, such as an EpiPen or inhaler, to address allergies or respiratory conditions during outdoor activities. opt for first aid kits that cater to your specific needs and conditions, and consider features such as adjustable compartments, waterproof materials, or other accessories that can enhance their functionality during outdoor activities.

Satellite Messenger or Personal Locator Beacon: Select a satellite messenger or personal locator beacon that can communicate with emergency services or loved ones during extended outdoor excursions. opt for devices that offer reliable coverage, long battery life, and other features that can enhance their functionality during outdoor activities, and ensure that they meet safety standards and regulations for outdoor activities.

Portable Water Filter or Purification System: Invest in a portable water filter or purification system to treat water from natural sources during long-term wilderness survival situations. opt for filters or purification systems that cater to your specific needs and conditions, and consider features such as flow rate, filtration efficiency, or other accessories that can enhance their functionality during outdoor activities.

Additional Preparations for Special Considerations and Eventualities: In addition to specialized equipment, consider additional preparations for special considerations and eventualities, such as:

Conducting a thorough risk assessment and developing a contingency plan before embarking on your excursion

Implementing proper safety measures, such as using safety harnesses, life vests, or other protective gear

Providing ample training and education to yourself and your companions on addressing unique scenarios during outdoor activities

Testing and Familiarization: Test and familiarize yourself with your special considerations and eventualities equipment before embarking on your outdoor excursion. Understand their functionality, adjustability, and other key features to ensure that you can effectively utilize them during your adventure and address any unique scenarios that may arise during your wilderness adventures.

When prepping for your outdoor adventure with special considerations and eventualities, carefully consider the selection, functionality, and testing of your additional equipment. By incorporating these devices into your prepping equipment kit, you can address unique scenarios, maintain safety and comfort.

Summary

Outdoor survival living requires careful planning, preparation, and the right equipment to ensure safety, comfort, and success. By considering essential tools and gadgets for navigation, fire and heat production, water and hygiene, food and nutrition, security and protection, first aid and medical supplies, power and lighting, and special considerations, you can be better prepared to tackle the challenges and joys of outdoor adventure.

Building a comprehensive outdoor survival kit takes time, research, and investment. Prioritize high-quality, lightweight, and versatile items that cater to your specific needs and preferences. Ensure you have a solid understanding of proper usage, maintenance, and storage for each piece of equipment.

Furthermore, consider enrolling in first aid and survival training courses to enhance your knowledge and skills. Practice using your equipment in controlled environments and gradually build your confidence and proficiency in various outdoor scenarios.

Finally, remember that the ultimate goal of outdoor survival living is not only about surviving but also about connecting with nature, fostering personal growth, and creating unforgettable memories. Embrace the journey, stay adaptable, and enjoy the adventure.